Freedom from

The Real Cause and Proven Self-Healing Plan

How I Found Relief When Nothing Else Worked

Isabella White

Disclaimer

The information in this book is based on the author's research, opinions, and experiences. It is not intended to replace professional medical advice or treatment. The reader should regularly consult a physician for any health issues and always seek the advice of a physician before modifying diet, supplement, or exercise regimens. The author and publisher shall have neither liability nor responsibility to any person or entity concerning any loss or damage related to the information contained in this book. The information provided is general and may not apply to every individual. Any reliance on the information contained herein is solely at the reader's risk.

Contents

Chapter 4

Introduction

It all started about two years ago, on a regular Wednesday morning. I had just finished my usual breakfast of oatmeal and fruit when an all-too-common pain hit me in the lower left side of my abdomen. I immediately knew I was in for yet another diverticulitis flare-up.

For those unfamiliar, diverticulitis occurs when small pouches called diverticula in the colon become infected and inflamed. It leads to intense abdominal pain, nausea, vomiting, fever, and chills. I had experienced several diverticulitis attacks before, but this one felt different—more severe and intense than usual.

After toughing it out at home for a day, the pain became unbearable. I couldn't eat or sleep; there was blood in my stool, and I was utterly exhausted from the nonstop vomiting. My wife finally convinced me to go to the emergency room. After several tests, scans, and hours of agonizing waiting, I was officially diagnosed with another type of acute diverticulitis.

The ER doctor said this was a particularly nasty flare-up that would require a multi-day hospital stay for IV antibiotics, bowel rest, and monitoring. I dreaded the thought of being cooped up in a hospital bed for days on end, not to mention the crazy medical bills headed my way. But I didn't have much choice, given the severity of the infection.

As I settled into the sterile hospital room, I felt defeated. It seemed like every time my diverticulitis symptoms finally subsided, and I started feeling better, another flare-up would eventually rear its ugly head. It was an endless cycle of pain and frustration. I was beyond tired of this chronic condition disrupting my life. But for now, as the IV dripped antibiotics into my veins, all I could do was rest and hope this hospital stay would get me back on my feet again. Diverticulitis was a battle, but I wasn't ready to surrender.

Chapter 1

What is Diverticulitis, and Why Was it Ruining My Life?

Anatomy of Diverticulitis and How it Develops

Diverticulitis begins with the formation of diverticula. These small, bulging pouches push outward from weak spots in the colon's wall. They form most commonly in the sigmoid colon, the last section of the colon before the rectum.

Diverticula start as tiny herniations in the muscular layer of the colon wall. They push through the weak areas where blood vessels penetrate the barrier. Pressure from gas and stools within the colon causes the pouches to expand. Over time, diverticula can grow up to several centimeters in size.

It's thought that abnormal colon motility and high pressure contribute to the development of diverticula. Stools moving too slowly through the colon increase pressure on the walls. Diets low in fiber and high in red meat may also increase the likelihood of developing diverticula. Smoking has been linked to a higher risk as well.

Generally, the presence of diverticula does not cause problems. About 80% of people with diverticula remain asymptomatic. However, issues arise when diverticula become obstructed, inflamed, or infected. Fecal matter and bacteria can become trapped within the pouches, causing swelling and infection.

This leads to diverticulitis, which is inflammation of the diverticula. It occurs when infections take hold within the swollen pouches. The body's immune response triggers inflammation to fight the disease. Blood and pus may collect in the affected diverticula.

Symptoms of a diverticulitis flare include intense abdominal pain, fever, nausea, vomiting, chills, and changes in bowel habits. A perforation can lead to a severe infection spilling into the abdominal cavity. Abscesses may also form adjacent to the affected diverticula.

Recurring bouts of acute diverticulitis can lead to chronic diverticulitis with ongoing inflammation and complications. Stopping the cycle requires identifying and avoiding triggers, diet changes, antibiotics, and possibly surgery if attacks are frequent. Detecting diverticulitis in its early stages is crucial for preventing it from significantly affecting one's quality of life.

The Standard and Debilitating Symptoms I Experienced with Diverticulitis

The first sign of an impending diverticulitis flare-up for me is usually a dull ache in my lower left abdomen. As the hours pass, the ache crescendos into unrelenting, piercing pain localized in that area. This extreme abdominal pain is the most prominent and debilitating symptom for me.

When a bout hits, the abdominal pain becomes so severe and unrelenting that I can focus on little else. Any movement or shifting exacerbates the stabbing sensation. I cannot find any relief, no matter what position I try. Even light pressure on the area, from clothing or a seatbelt, for example, is excruciating. The intense pain makes it impossible to function normally. All I can do is remain motionless until it passes.

In addition to agonizing abdominal pain, nausea, and vomiting frequently accompany my diverticulitis flares. The vomiting causes painful spasms in my inflamed colon. I break out in cold, clammy sweats as my body tries to fight the infection. On several occasions, I became so dehydrated from nonstop vomiting that I required hospitalization for IV fluid replacement.

Low-grade fever and chills are also common for me during an acute attack. My temperature usually hovers around 100–101 °F. The colds cause my teeth to chatter uncontrollably. I pile on blankets to try and get warm, but the chills refuse to subside until the flare has run its course.

Losing my appetite is another typical symptom. When I am experiencing an episode, the mere thought of food is repulsive. I'm unable to keep down anything besides small sips of clear liquids until the nausea passes. My body is deprived of nutrients, which causes weakness and fatigue.

In addition to the crippling pain and digestive distress, diverticulitis flares take a huge mental and emotional toll. The fear of when the next flare will strike always lurks in the back of my mind between episodes. The chronic nature of this condition and the repeatedly derailed plans are incredibly frustrating and disheartening. But the pain itself remains the worst part by far.

Conventional Treatment Failures and Frustrations I Experienced

When I first started having diverticulitis flare-ups, my doctor's advice was usually the same: a liquid diet and oral antibiotics to treat the infection. However, as the episodes became more frequent, this conventional treatment approach proved largely ineffective for me.

The antibiotics would provide some short-term relief for my symptoms when taken at the onset of a flare. However, time and again, the diverticulitis would return as soon as I finished the prescription. It was incredibly frustrating to deal with the same painful symptoms over and over. The antibiotics were not resolving the underlying condition.

I worked closely with my gastroenterologist to identify trigger foods and adjust my diet to prevent recurrences. Removing nuts, seeds, corn, and other foods aggravating diverticula provided some benefits. But despite my diligent dietary changes, I still experienced too many flares.

When attacks did strike, I was reluctant to turn to antibiotics each time immediately. I worried about building resistance with repeated use. And since oral antibiotics alone were not giving me lasting relief anyway, I hesitated to go through yet another round of medication with unpleasant side effects.

Several severe episodes required hospitalization for intravenous antibiotics and bowel rest. But again, the treatment would only provide temporary improvement. Once discharged, it felt like just a matter of time before the familiar pain would return. The cycle of antibiotics, short-term relief, and then recurrence was draining both physically and emotionally.

I became more and more disheartened by the absence of long-lasting solutions. Despite adhering well to conventional medical advice, I experienced a significant reduction in the quality of my life. My gastroenterologist suggested scheduling colonoscopy procedures after each flare-up to monitor for complications. While essential, colonoscopies themselves cause discomfort without fixing the underlying problem.

The traditional treatment path was not giving me adequate control over my diverticulitis. I needed more than just temporary pain relief and monitoring. I wanted my life back for good. That motivation pushed me to expand my search for treatments beyond conventional medicine alone. There had to be better options out there.

Chapter 2

Identifying the Root Cause

After yet another miserable hospitalization for diverticulitis, I decided it was time to dig deeper into the root cause of why I kept experiencing recurrent flare-ups. There had to be more to it than just the presence of diverticula in my colon. I wanted to understand what was driving the ongoing inflammation and infection.

In my research, I learned more about our gut microbiome's critical role in digestive health and immunity. The microbiome consists of trillions of bacteria, viruses, and fungi that live symbiotically in the gastrointestinal tract. This complex ecosystem, also known as dysbiosis, can quickly become thrown off balance.

The Gut Microbiome and How an Imbalance Can Cause Inflammation

The gut microbiome is a complex community of microorganisms living in our intestines. This includes hundreds of bacterial species, viruses, fungi, and other microbes. A healthy gut has diverse beneficial bacteria to keep everything balanced.

The microbiome is critical for many bodily functions, from metabolism and nutrition absorption to immune response and inflammation regulation. The beneficial bacteria help digest fiber, make vitamins, prevent infection, and keep pathogenic species in check. A harmonious microbiome equals good health.

Dysbiosis occurs when an imbalance in the microbiome and harmful bacteria take over. Antibiotics, poor diet, chronic stress, and illnesses can wipe out the good bacteria and allow nasty bugs to flourish. Dysbiosis causes the microbiome to act abnormally, initiating widespread effects.

With dysbiosis, excessive gram-negative bacteria produce endotoxins that trigger the body's immune defenses. This stimulates chronic, low-grade inflammation as a reaction. Inflammatory chemicals called cytokines are released systemically, causing damage when uncontrolled.

Inflammation is meant to be a short-term response to injury or infection. However, dysbiosis can cause a nonstop inflammatory state that contributes to disease. Various health conditions, from autoimmune disorders to depression, have been linked to prolonged inflammation stemming from the gut.

Additionally, the out-of-balance microbiome has difficulty maintaining the intestinal lining. A compromised gut barrier allows bacteria, toxins, and undigested food particles to escape the intestines and enter the bloodstream. Intestinal permeability, or "leaky gut," further drives inflammation.

When it came to my recurrent diverticulitis, antibiotics and a high-stress lifestyle likely disrupted my microbiome over time, leading to dysbiosis. The resulting inflammation created an environment ripe for ongoing infection and complications in my colon.

By addressing the root cause of the gut imbalance fueling the fire, I hoped to calm the downstream inflammation wreaking havoc in my body. Rebalancing my microbiome became essential to resolving my health issues.

The Link Between Diet, Stress, Lifestyle Factors, and Diverticulitis

For many years, experts believed a low-fiber diet primarily caused diverticulitis. More recent research indicates the role of diet and other lifestyle factors is more complex. Things like chronic stress and poor sleep may contribute just as much, if not more, to diverticulitis flare-ups.

There is a strong connection between the development of diverticula pouches and one's dietary habits. A low-fiber diet can lead to constipation and increased pressure on the colon walls. This may cause small herniations of the diverticula over time. Diets high in red meat and fat versus plant foods are also associated with greater risk.

However, diet alone does not determine which people with diverticulitis go on to struggle with repeated bouts of diverticulitis. Many asymptomatic individuals eat similar diets to those with recurrent diverticulitis. This indicates other factors are likely involved in the progression of the disease.

Stress may play a primary role in altering gut function and microbiome balance. Diverticulitis flares often follow periods of high pressure. Stress hormones can impact stomach acid production, intestinal mobility, inflammation, and protective mucus production. All of these effects may promote diverticulitis.

A chronic lack of sleep is problematic as well. Poor sleep is linked to increased inflammation and insulin resistance. Insulin helps regulate anti-inflammatory gut bacteria, so insulin disruption promotes further inflammation. Sleep deprivation also suppresses immune function, raising infection susceptibility.

Regular exercise helps reduce visceral fat, which secretes pro-inflammatory hormones. Obesity leads to more systemic inflammation that could influence diverticulitis risk. Smoking and excessive alcohol intake are other lifestyle habits shown to impact gut health negatively.

In my case, high stress levels and sleep deprivation were likely significant contributors to my recurrent diverticulitis battles. My hectic work schedule and worries over flare-ups created a vicious cycle. Dietary and other lifestyle tweaks helped, but learning stress management techniques became just as critical for breaking the cycle of flares.

Note: No single factor determines diverticulitis susceptibility. To progress from asymptomatic to recurrent diverticulitis in those who are genetically predisposed, an individualized, multifactorial approach is required. Factors such as diet, exercise, stress, alcohol use, smoking, and sleep play a role.

Specific Triggers Disrupting my Gut Health

After analyzing my lifestyle and health history, a few key triggers stood out that likely contributed to my battles with repeated diverticulitis flare-ups.

First, chronic stress was probably public enemy number one when it came to disrupting my gut health. My high-pressure job had me in a constant state of anxiety. Worrying about work issues consumed my thoughts in the evenings and on weekends. This resulted in elevated cortisol and systemic inflammation that predisposed me to gut issues.

Additionally, my diet was higher in inflammatory foods and lower in beneficial fiber than ideal. I ate a lot of processed foods for convenience, including lunch meats that contain nitrates. My vegetable intake was minimal. These dietary factors promoted an imbalanced gut microbiome and intestinal inflammation.

Lack of regular exercise also didn't help matters. I spent most days sitting at a desk with little time for movement or activity. Increased visceral abdominal fat and bodywide inflammation from sedentary behavior likely made me more susceptible to diverticulitis flares.

Sleep was another problem area. I regularly slept less than 6 hours per night. My mind would race about work stressors when I lay down to sleep. Sleep deprivation adds to the issues by impairing immune function and fueling inflammation.

Finally, recurring antibiotic use was probably the nail in the coffin when it came to crippling my gut health. While necessary for treating acute infections, long-term overuse of antibiotics likely decimated populations of beneficial bacteria in my gut over time. This allowed more harmful and inflammatory species to dominate.

Chronic stress, an inflammatory diet, inactivity, lack of sleep, and overuse of antibiotics created the perfect gut health storm. This cascade of effects threw my microbiome totally out of balance and primed me for repeated bouts of misery. As such, improving my lifestyle habits and gut function became paramount to overcoming diverticulitis.

Chapter 3

My Proven 4-Step Plan to Heal My Gut and Beat Diverticulitis

After years of frustration and false starts, I finally developed an effective 4-step plan to resolve my ongoing struggles with diverticulitis. My gut health and quality of life have vastly improved by working through these steps:

Step 1: Adopting an Anti-Inflammatory and Diverticulitis-Friendly Diet

The first critical step was overhauling my diet to be rich in gut-soothing foods yet gentle on the colon. With the help of a nutritionist, I devised a diverticulitis diet plan focused on reducing inflammation and optimizing digestion. Key changes included:

1. **Eliminating Problem Foods:** I cut out inflammatory triggers like fried foods, fatty red meat, processed carbs, excess sugar, and alcohol. I also avoided common diverticulitis aggravators like nuts, seeds, popcorn, and corn. This calmed the irritation and made flare-ups less likely.

2. **Eating More Plants:** I substantially increased plant-based foods full of soluble fiber like oats, leafy greens, squash, beans, artichokes, berries, and non-citrus fruits. The fiber feeds beneficial bacteria and keeps the bowels regular. Eating a wide variety of produce also increases antioxidant and phytonutrient intake to fight inflammation.

3. **Choosing Healthy Proteins:** My protein sources shifted from red meat to wild-caught fish and organic poultry, plus plant proteins like legumes, nuts, seeds, and tofu. Cold-water fish provide anti-inflammatory omega-3s. I also used spices like turmeric, ginger, and garlic, which have anti-inflammatory properties.

4. **Staying Hydrated:** I aimed for at least 64 ounces of fluids daily, mainly in herbal tea, water with lemon, and diluted fruit juices. Proper hydration prevents constipation and keeps things moving smoothly through the colon to avoid irritation of the diverticula pouches.

5. **Timing Meals Wisely:** I started eating smaller, frequent meals every 3–4 hours rather than 1-2 giant meals daily. This prevents pressure buildup in the

colon. I also avoided food 3 hours before bedtime to allow thorough digestion before lying down.

These evidence-based dietary tweaks formed the foundation for reducing intestinal inflammation, optimizing gut health, and preventing recurrent diverticulitis flares. It took dedication, but the effort paid off tremendously in improving my quality of life.

Step 2: Managing Stress and Anxiety with Diverticulitis-Safe Techniques

Once the diet was addressed, I focused Step 2 on stress management and mental well-being. My doctor advised avoiding intense core abdominal exercises during active diverticulitis flares. So, I implemented several safe, low-impact mind-body practices:

1. **Yoga:** I followed gentle, restorative yoga routines relying on supported poses rather than intense core engagement. These focused on relaxation, stretching, and deep breathing. Twists and hip openers are calming and great for digestion.

2. **Meditation:** Sitting upright, I did short, 10-15 minute guided meditations once or twice daily. Meditating reduced my anxiety and cortisol levels,

promoting intestinal healing. I used apps like Calm for diverse meditations.

3. **Breathing Exercises:** Taking 5–10 minutes for deep belly breathing gave me a quick stress-relief boost any time of day. Inhaling deeply through the nose and exhaling fully relaxed my nervous system.

4. **Mindfulness:** I tapped into mindfulness by staying present during simple daily activities like brushing my teeth, washing dishes, and walking the dog. This diffused my fixation on past worries or future anxieties.

5. **Nature Therapy:** Getting outside daily provides mood-boosting benefits and health-promoting microbiome diversity through environmental microbe exposures. A short neighborhood walk or sitting outside assured me I got fresh air.

6. **Aromatherapy:** Smelling pleasant, calming essential oils like lavender helped reduce stress. Diffusing oils or applying diluted oil to pulse points offered quick relaxation.

7. **Massage:** I booked therapeutic massages that lowered cortisol and calmed the vagus nerve that controls gut function. But even a brief self-massage helped.

8. **Sleep:** Getting on an earlier sleep schedule and limiting electronics before bed drastically improved my sleep quality. This gave my mind and body time to recharge.

Engaging in these gut-safe relaxation techniques became vital for breaking the chronic stress-intestinal inflammation connection fueling my diverticulitis flares. Managing stress and anxiety simultaneously with diet optimized my results long-term.

Step 3: Optimizing Gut Health with Targeted Supplements and Probiotics

Step 3 of my plan focused on specific supplements to reduce inflammation, repair the intestinal lining, and rebalance my gut microbiome after recurrent antibiotics battered it. Essential supplements I relied on included:

- Probiotics with at least 25–50 billion CFUs are rotated weekly between formulas with lactobacilli, bifidobacteria, and soil-based species like Bacillus subtilis. Restoring microbial diversity was crucial.
- Prebiotics like acacia fiber, inulin, and arabinogalactans feed probiotics and enhance their

efficacy. Getting prebiotic-soluble fibers from food sources was also a priority.

- Glutamine powder is provided at 5–10 grams per day to fuel intestinal cell repair and regeneration of gut barrier tissue. Preventing "leaky gut" stops systemic inflammation from endotoxins escaping the intestines.

- Quercetin offers anti-inflammatory and antioxidant support, 500–1000 mg daily. It calms the immune response and inhibits the production of inflammatory cytokines.

- Curcumin enhances quercetin absorption. I took 500 mg of curcumin with 5–10 mg of piperine daily. Curcumin has similar anti-inflammatory mechanisms as quercetin.

- Zinc, at 30mg daily, boosts immune health and cell regeneration. Zinc is vital for microbiome balance and intestinal tissue repair.

- Vitamin D as microencapsulated D3, 4000-5000 IU daily, modulates immune activity and controls inflammation pathways. Vitamin D also improves bacterial composition in the gut.

Timing supplementation properly was critical. I took probiotics on an empty stomach and prebiotics with meals.

The glutamine and zinc I used at night to optimize healing during sleep. My practitioner adjusted dosages over time based on follow-up testing.

A mix of targeted nutrients and microbiome-rebalancing probiotics significantly improved my gut lining, controlled inflammation, and prevented recurrent infection and dysfunction.

Step 4: Maintaining a Healthy Lifestyle and Tuning Into My Body's Signals

After addressing my root causes through diet, stress management, and strategic supplementation, Step 4 was about sustaining the lifestyle changes long-term. Keeping inflammation down required diligence, even during periods when I felt well. Key aspects included:

1. **Exercise:** I aimed for at least 30 minutes of moderate exercise, like walking or swimming, five days per week. Exercise reduces visceral fat, boosts circulation, and increases microbiome diversity. I listened to my body and avoided intense activity during flares.

2. **Sleep:** Sticking to a consistent sleep routine was crucial for keeping cortisol and inflammation in

check. I went to bed at the same time every night and avoided screens before bed. Adequate sleep gave my body time to heal.

3. **Hydration:** Drinking adequate water and herbal tea daily prevents constipation and supports healthy elimination. Staying hydrated maintains electrolyte balance, too.

4. **Mindfulness:** Continuing daily meditation, deep breathing, and yoga grounded me in the present—this relieved stress and anxiety between diverticulitis episodes.

5. **Dietary Balance:** I stuck to my anti-inflammatory diet 80% of the time. Allowing small treats 20% of the time made the program sustainable long-term without feeling deprived.

6. **Stress Relief:** Whether soaking in a bath, calling a friend, or taking a nature walk, I carved out time daily for self-care to manage stress. Protecting my peace of mind was non-negotiable.

7. **Body Awareness:** I tuned into subtle symptoms like slight abdominal discomfort that typically preceded total diverticulitis attacks. Watching for early warning signs lets me proactively tweak my diet and lifestyle to prevent significant flare-ups.

Staying vigilant about healthy habits, even when feeling my best, was critical to avoiding backslides. Consistency optimized my gut function and microbiome balance over many months. With an integrative approach and close self-monitoring, I successfully broke the cycle of repeat diverticulitis attacks.

Chapter 4

My Personal Journey to Freedom from Diverticulitis

Documenting My Implementation of the Plan and Road to Recovery

After my fourth hospitalization for diverticulitis, I finally committed fully to my integrative 4-step healing plan. I was determined to take control and end this frustrating cycle of flare-ups.

During the initial two months, my primary focus was making significant changes to my diet to achieve a healthier eating pattern and lifestyle. I removed all processed foods and inflammatory triggers, much to the concern of my family, who didn't initially understand this restrictive approach. But when my pain and diarrhea resolved quickly, they became supportive.

Sticking to my diet while traveling for work posed challenges. I had to get creative, packing nuts and fruits and prepared meals in my suitcase. Saying no to happy hours and client dinners was difficult professionally but necessary for my health.

Meanwhile, I began doing yoga, meditation, and breathing exercises daily to reduce stress. This provided tremendous anxiety relief and improved my sleep quality. I felt more mentally resilient to handle work pressures without internalizing constant worry.

After about three months, I started taking strategic supplements under my doctor's guidance. I slowly added each one to allow my body time to adjust. Getting used to swallowing so many pills took patience, but the impact on my gut health made it worthwhile.

Occasional mild diverticulitis symptoms still popped up during the first six months. But instead of spiraling into a major flare, the discomfort is resolved within a day or two with rest and herbal tea. I took it as proof that my microbiome was stabilizing.

It's now been over a year since I began my gut healing plan, and I've not had a severe diverticulitis attack requiring antibiotics or hospitalization. I have much more energy and zest for life. My family is amazed by my miraculous improvement.

While it took dedication, addressing the root causes of imbalance in my body and microbiome was the key. My four-pronged approach allowed me to heal instead of just temporarily managing symptoms. I'm so grateful to be free of diverticulitis's grip and feel like myself again. It takes consistency, but a fulfilling life is possible. My journey can inspire others!

Tips for Identifying and Preventing Trigger Foods

Keep a food and symptom journal. Track everything you eat and any symptoms you experience to uncover associations. Look for patterns linking specific foods to abdominal pain, bloating, nausea, etc.

1. **Try eliminating diets.** Eliminate suspect foods for 2-4 weeks, then reintroduce one at a time while monitoring symptoms for a flare-up. Common triggers to eliminate include nuts, seeds, corn, beans, cruciferous veggies, and fried or fatty foods.
2. **Listen to your body.** Pay attention to subtle signals like gas, constipation, or loose stools that may precede full-blown symptoms. Adjust your diet at the first sign of irritation.

3. **Go low on FODMAP.** Limiting fermentable carbohydrates through a low-FODMAP diet can rest the colon and identify triggers. Reintroduce high-FODMAP foods slowly.

4. **Practice portion control.** Even safe foods can provoke symptoms if overeaten. Be mindful of portions to avoid putting excess pressure on the colon.

5. **Chew thoroughly.** Breaking food down mechanically through careful chewing reduces work for the colon.

6. **Stay hydrated.** Drink adequate fluids daily to keep the bowels regular. Dehydration aggravates constipation.

7. **Manage stress.** High stress is a common attack trigger. Keep stress in check through lifestyle changes and relaxation techniques.

8. **Consider food sensitivity testing.** Testing can detect sensitivities contributing to inflammation. Common culprits include gluten, dairy, and eggs.

Maintaining a healthy diet and lifestyle is vital to prevent recurrent diverticulitis flares, even during symptom-free periods.

Tips for Coping with Occasional Minor Flare-ups of Diverticulitis Symptoms

1. **Rest.** Get extra rest and avoid strenuous activity that can worsen inflammation. Listen to your body's signals.

2. **Apply heat.** Place a heating pad or hot water bottle over your lower abdomen for 15-20 minutes to help ease spasms and pain.

3. **Try over-the-counter pain relievers.** Medications like acetaminophen or ibuprofen can help reduce discomfort when used sparingly.

4. **Adjust your diet.** Stick to a clear liquid diet and avoid solid foods during a flare. Limit fiber intake temporarily to give your colon a rest.

5. **Prevent dehydration.** Be sure to sip clear fluids like water, broth, and herbal tea throughout the day. Dehydration can exacerbate constipation.

6. **Consider sipping aloe juice.** The anti-inflammatory properties of aloe vera juice may aid healing during mild flares.

7. **Try soothing herbal teas.** Ginger, peppermint, chamomile, and fennel teas can help settle digestive distress.

8. **Take probiotics.** Continue probiotics to support your gut microbiome balance; avoid prebiotics that feed bacteria.

9. **Manage stress.** Employ relaxation techniques like deep breathing, meditation, or music therapy to curb stress.

10. **Know when to call your doctor.** Seek medical advice if symptoms persist beyond 2–3 days or suddenly worsen. Don't hesitate to be evaluated.

Most minor flares can be managed at home with conservative symptom relief measures. It is important to remain vigilant about any changes and seek medical attention.

Motivational Advice to Fellow Diverticulitis Sufferers Based on My Experience

I know the battle with diverticulitis can feel lonely and frustrating at times. The flares and abdominal pain take a substantial physical and emotional toll. It's easy to get discouraged when symptoms keep recurring, no matter what you try. But there is hope!

Healing is a process. Making even small diet and lifestyle changes builds momentum. Be patient and kind to yourself.

Progress will come in fits and starts, but stay consistent. Experiment to find what works specifically for your body; no one-size-fits-all approach exists.

This condition does not define you. Don't let diverticulitis dominate your self-identity and steal your joy. You are still the same wonderful person with much to offer. Let your hopes and dreams motivate you through tough days.

Remember, you are not alone. Millions suffer from diverticulitis and understand the daily struggles. Connect with others who get it for support and advice. Just sharing your experience can help someone else feel less alone.

Most importantly, don't give up hope. There are many paths to healing if you advocate for yourself and stay determined. New treatments emerge all the time. You can regain control of your health, even when progress feels slow. Have faith that you can break free of this condition and thrive. I believe in you!

Conclusion

If you're struggling with repeated bouts of miserable diverticulitis, I hope my journey offers some guidance and inspiration. This debilitating condition does not have to define your life. Lasting relief is within reach with consistent effort and a personalized, root-cause-based approach.

Remember, recurrent diverticulitis often stems from an underlying gut imbalance fueling chronic inflammation; identifying and addressing your specific triggers, whether dietary, lifestyle-related, or otherwise, is critical. Be patient and keep tweaking your individualized plan until you find what moves the needle.

Supporting overall health should be the goal, not just temporarily minimizing diverticulitis symptoms when they strike. With the right combination of lifestyle changes, stress management, dietary strategies, targeted supplements, and advanced testing, you can break the cycle for good.

Stay motivated through ups and downs by focusing on your vision for health and happiness. Be kind to yourself through this process. It takes time to heal after years of recurrence. But have faith that you will find your perfect path if you stay on the course.

You are stronger than you know. Don't allow diverticulitis to steal one more day from you. The power is within you to regain control of your gut health, end inflammation at its roots, and live fully again. Keep fighting! You can be one of the many diverticulitis success stories with courage and persistence.

My parting words: believe in your ability to heal and transform your health. Stay focused on the bright future ahead. Better days are coming if you keep moving forward with purpose and passion. You've got this! Now, empower yourself and others by sharing your journey.

Appendix

Meal Plans, Recipes, and Food Lists

7-Day Anti-Inflammatory Meal Plan

Day 1	**Breakfast:** Avocado toast with poached egg, tomato, spinach
	Lunch: Greek yogurt, mixed berries, slivered almonds
	Dinner: Baked salmon, quinoa, and roasted broccoli
	Snack: Carrots and hummus
Day 2	**Breakfast:** Oatmeal with walnuts, cinnamon, and blueberries
	Lunch: Lentil vegetable soup
	Dinner: Chicken stir-fry with cauliflower rice
	Snack: Apple slices with nut butter
Day 3	**Breakfast:** Veggie frittata
	Lunch: Tuna salad with lettuce wraps

	Dinner: Turkey meatballs, zucchini noodles, marinara sauce
	Snack: Smoothie with banana, spinach, and almond milk
Day 4	**Breakfast:** Chia seed pudding with almond milk and strawberries
	Lunch: Grilled chicken spinach salad
	Dinner: Portobello mushroom burgers on whole-grain buns
	Snack: Hardboiled eggs
Day 5	**Breakfast:** Overnight oats with chia seeds, cinnamon, and almond milk
	Lunch: Salmon salad stuffed with tomatoes
	Dinner: Sheet pan-roasted vegetables and chicken sausage
	Snack: Cucumber slices with cottage cheese
Day 6	**Breakfast:** Vegetable egg scramble
	Lunch: Chicken rice bowl with avocado
	Dinner: Hearty vegetable soup

	Snack: Rice cakes with smoked salmon and cream cheese
Day 7	**Breakfast:** Nut granola with Greek yogurt and fruit
	Lunch: Quinoa tabbouleh salad
	Dinner: Grilled shrimp and vegetable kebabs
	Snack: Trail mix with nuts, seeds, and coconut

Anti-Inflammatory Recipes:

1. Gut-Soothing Chicken Noodle Soup
2. Mediterranean Tuna Salad
3. Overnight Chia Seed Oatmeal
4. Salmon Avocado Bowl
5. Roasted Root Vegetables
6. Berry Coconut Smoothie
7. Turkey Lettuce Wraps
8. Chickpea and Kale Stew

Recommended Food List:

Proteins:	Salmon, tuna, chicken, turkey, eggs, plant-based protein powder
Fruits:	Berries, citrus, pineapple, grapes, apples, and pears
Vegetables:	Leafy greens, cruciferous veggies (cooked), carrots, squash
Grains:	Oats, brown rice, quinoa, and buckwheat
Legumes:	Lentils, chickpeas, beans
Nuts and seeds:	Almonds, walnuts, chia, flaxseed
Oils/Fats:	Olive oil, avocado oil, coconut oil, avocados
Beverages:	Green tea, herbal tea, lemon water, chilled peppermint tea
Spices:	Turmeric, ginger, garlic, rosemary, thyme, oregano, cinnamon

Made in the USA
Columbia, SC
07 December 2024